The Breaking of Me

Lisa Scovell-Strickland

MY HEART

Delicate like a strand of silk
More precious than the crown jewels
My heart beats within my breast
Its love knows no bounds
Its pain echoes through each vein
Handle with care
Caress at every opportunity
For when it breaks
The pieces will scatter to the ends of the earth

First Published in 2024 by
Stone Phoenix Press in collaboration with Lemon Jelly Press
Isle of Wight
UK
PO36 0LL

Copyright lies with the author.
All rights reserved. No part of this publication can be reproduced, stored in a retrieval system, or transmitted in any form or by any means, electronic, mechanical, photocopying, recoding or otherwise, without prior permission of the publishers.

This publication is sold subject to the condition that it shall not, by way of trade or otherwise, be lent, re-sold, hired out or otherwise circulated without the publisher's prior consent in any form of binding or cover other than that which it is published and without a similar condition including this condition being imposed on the subsequent purchaser.

ISBN 978-1-7395415-0-7
Cover design by Lisa Scovell-Strickland

Acknowledgements

There are many who have in one way or another contributed to the collection that you are about to read. However, I want to thank the best of them:

The Cameo Stranger once told me that, "behind your fear lies your truth and this is where we always need to go and seek". This collection is the embodiment of my fears and my truths. I thank them for their continuing support.

My beautiful wife Zara, thank you for your warm embrace where I feel safe even in my darkest moments. My love for you is an ardent flame which you fuel every day.

My chosen family, Annette, Darren, Emily and Olivia. I am grateful to have you all in my life.

My cheerleaders Charlotte, Claire, Debbie, Jazmine and Tracy, who have been there for me during the ups, the downs and everything in between. I thank you, my beautiful sisters.

I plugged the fracture in my heart with all the hurtful words you said / and the worst memories that you tried to etch into my skin / all I could hear within my heart were the poison penned letters that you wrote to me / along with the drop beats which were out of step with my natural rhythm / you tried to un-say the words, return them to your crooked mouth / but you cannot un-ring the bell and I cannot un-hear those words / So I am left bereft, looking at my fractured heart / hoping that it will not shatter completely / as I search inside myself to find something strong enough to bind these wounds / to make me feel whole again

FRACTURED

CONTENTS

THE BREAKING OF ME..1
DREAMING OF MY OWN FAIRYTALE......................2
WHEN THE DARKNESS CAME...................................3
WHEN THE DARKNESS DRAGS YOU DOWN...........4
WHERE MY GUILT WAS BORN....................................5
GUILT...6
JOY UNDERLINED BY GRIEF.......................................7
QUICK RELEASE..8
THERE IS A SPIDER ON MY CEILING........................9
EMPTINESS AND SORROW..10
FADING...11
STUCK...12
TODAY...13
SPIRALLING INTO OBLIVION..............................14-15
UNTITLED..16
ACCEPTANCE..17
FROM THE SEDUCED TO THE SEDUCER.............18
GHOSTED BY YOU..19
LAST DANCE...20
REFLECTIONS, REGRETS, REPOSE........................21
LEFT ON A READ RECEIPT..................................22-23
SUBMISSION...24
NOT MY OWN SELF...25
A CHANCE MEETING..26
MANSPLAINING..27
BLUES BAR RENDITION..28
PRESENT..29
DEAR..30-31
RELATIONSHIP GOALS...32

GOODBYE TO A LOYAL FRIEND	33
STALEMATE	34
THE WAY WE CONVERSE WITH EACH OTHER	35
HIDING FROM THE DARKNESS OF YOU	36-37
PROVOCATION	38
WAR PAINT	39
KEEPING MYSELF SAFE FROM THE DARKNESS OF YOU	40-41
HOW FAR I FELL INTO DARKNESS	42-43
NO SUITOR WAS RIGHT FOR ME	44-45
CRASH AND BURN	46-47
WHERE I HIDE MY TEARS	48
THE EVERLASTING TORMENT OF YOUR WORDS	49
WHEN THE WATER OVERWHELMED	50-51
STUCK	52
I KNEW THAT THE DARKNESS WAS BACK	53
CHEMICAL SUBMISSION	54
UP AND DOWN, AGAIN AND AGAIN	55
BREAKING FREE OF THE DARKNESS ONCE MORE	56-57
THE DARKNESS HAUNTS ME STILL	58-59
THE BITTER TASTE OF SLEEP	60
HAPPENSTANCE NO MORE	61
THE GHOST IN THE HALLWAY MIRROR	62
THE WORDS IN MY HEAD	63
AFTER THE WORLD REOPENED	64-65
THE BATHROOM MIRROR CRACKED	66-67
EXHAUSTION	68-69
IN BETWEEN	70-71

THE BREAKING OF ME

It didn't happen suddenly
I didn't fall and break into pieces
It was a slow process
The bindings winding tighter with each breath I took
Each word cutting finely over and over
My body starting to betray me

Anxiety spiraling my mind
Twisting my gut in upon itself
My limbs heavy with sorrow
My tongue thick with emotion
So much so that I couldn't swallow
Choking on my attempts to ask for help

When I truly realised that I was shattered into a million pieces
I could hardly recognise myself

A ghost in the mirror
A shadow in the light
Small and insignificant

Hoping I would rise again
Transforming into something new
Something strong and beautiful

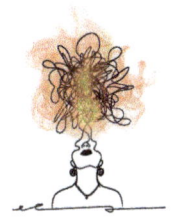

DREAMING OF MY OWN FAIRYTALE

I remember when I first knew that I was different
That my story wouldn't be a traditional fairytale
It was the summer at the peak of my childhood
And whilst other girls were re-enacting their traditional gender roles
I didn't want to be the princess who kissed a frog and married a prince
I wanted to be the princess who fought the dragon to save the other princess

But I couldn't play this role
I couldn't say these words aloud
For the fear of being different was suffocating

So, I played the homemaker, the wife who takes care of her husband
Preparing myself for the reality that was yet to come
But dreaming of my fairytale where the princess fought and won

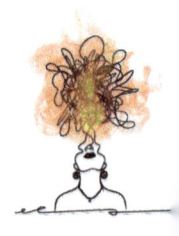

WHEN THE DARKNESS CAME

I remember when the darkness first invaded my senses
The tendrils seeped in through my pores and clung to the very fibre of me

I wondered why sadness kept its grip on me
Why all my colours faded to monochrome
Why the joy I had always carried was slowly ripped from my soul

I clawed at myself desperate to get it out at first
As time went on, realisation struck that this wouldn't be temporary

I would have to learn to manage this as best I could
I tried to find the source
Hoped I could snuff it out
But it wouldn't be that easy

So I prepared myself for a war
Within which I would fight myself
Against myself
To find myself once more

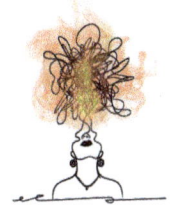

WHEN THE DARKNESS DRAGS YOU DOWN

Today feels like I am wading through mud
Up to my waist and clinging on to anything for dear life

Each step I take painful and slow
My ankles fighting to lift my feet
My knees screaming at the weight that they are carrying

From the waist up the struggle doesn't show
As I stretch out to ease my shoulders
But with each step the mud gets deeper
Dragging me to the bottom where the darkness hides

It will only be satisfied when it has all of me

So I reach up, arms outstretched
Hoping that someone realises I'm in trouble
To throw me a lifeline and pull me to safety

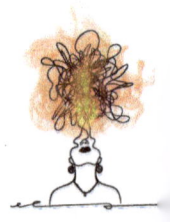

WHERE MY GUILT WAS BORN

That shame of what I did will never leave me
I cannot take it back
My actions from the outside appeared selfish
From where I stood I was just trying to stop the pain
Dull it into submission so I could breathe easy again
As I tried to dull the pain with each swallow
I slowly counted each one down

As I got to ten I realised this wasn't what I wanted
I didn't want that finality
I just wanted it all to stop and give me peace
I just wanted to be me and loved for who I was
I wanted to know love
I wanted to have a future where I was accepted
So I begged my hands to stop
I replaced the cap

Knowing that tomorrow I would have to confess all my sins
Knowing that there would be an interrogation
Knowing that I would have to fight for myself again and again
That that fight would cleave me in two
That I would forever have to atone for what I had done
That I would always have to fight for myself
Hoping that one day that I could be myself
Even if I had to carry the guilt and shame forever more

GUILT

I stand alone, weighted down, a heavy burden on my shoulders
Strapped in place around my heart
That sagging feeling slowing me down
Keeping me rooted to the spot
Now immobile, caught in my own trap
It is the weight of all my guilt
Braced with shame, wrapped in fear
Laced with a sprinkle of self-loathing

It all prevents me from progress, from reaching my goals
From mending broken bridges
From healing me within
As I replay those actions I took
As I whisper those words exchanged
Despite my best efforts, I cannot wipe my slate clean

So, I bear the guilt as best I can
Hoping that the weight will gradually subside
Trying not to add more to the pile
Wishing I could have made better choices

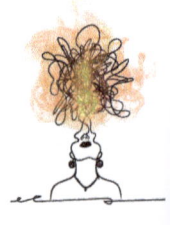

JOY UNDERLINED BY GRIEF

I met your precious new joy today
So perfect, innocent, tiny
I swore to protect her forever
Whilst a poisoned arrow pierced me deep

The tip angled to reopen old wounds
The dream of what I wanted most festers

My eyes tighten with a pain once dulled
I hear the shattering of me at once

I cling to how happy you are in this moment
I am overjoyed for you

But I am underlined by an inconsolable grief
Of what for me was never meant to be

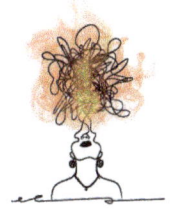

QUICK RELEASE

It sleeps and silence fills my thoughts
Deep passions dwell within
But once it wakes, I start to sip the potent mood
Swirling desires stir within
Feelings controlled no longer in its wake
From deep within, it grows
It rises slowly in me, I feel giddy at its pleasure
Within me comes desires untold
Tasting the sweetness of desire, it feeds
Desires, passions out of control, within
It feeds on fear, revels in the pain it causes
All control comes from within
Pain in fear, life in love and so the desires get stronger
Consumed I listen within
Finally free I wish it had always been like this
My secret from within momentary but endless

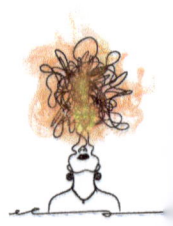

THERE IS A SPIDER ON MY CEILING

There is a spider on the ceiling, looking down at me

There is a spider on my ceiling, staring at me with glee

There is a spider on my ceiling, sauntering my way

There is a spider on my ceiling, what will she have to say

There is a spider on my ceiling, she starts to spin her web

There is a spider on my ceiling, getting into my head

There is a spider on my ceiling, I am caught in her trap

There is a spider on my ceiling, I feel my mettle snap

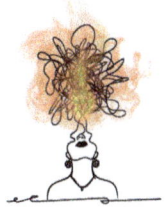

EMPTINESS AND SORROW

Shattered moments and bittersweet dreams
Another insomnia pill for me
Every time sleep fills my being, I dread
The thought of who I will be some day
Trevor never said it would be easy
I struggle on and try to wish the night away
The long dark good night looms over
Waiting for me to drop my guard
Only my memories can save me now
As the stars conspire against us all

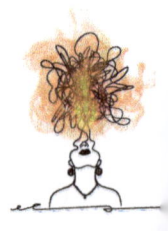

FADING

Lipstick smudged
Eyes blurred
Another great party
Self-esteem high
Blood at boiling point
Yet another night, not in an empty bed

Dressed to kill every night
A chain of forgotten lovers
Kiss and tell tomorrow
Leaving yourself an open void
Why carry on this game?
Don't do this to yourself

Justifications paled in reputation
Whispers too often unkind
You hold your head high
Do you really feel that good inside?
Is it an addiction? Is there a cure?
Do you know that you are fading?

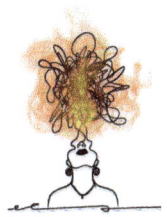

STUCK

Trapped in a cardboard box sealed from the inside
Only looking out in Sunday best
How drole everyday life is
The little things that amuse us
Now disgust me to the very core
Boredom sets in as the bats
Take up residence in the belfry
I need work soon otherwise I shall be
Lost within my own thoughts
A maze too complex I'd lose myself
Within myself once more
I scream

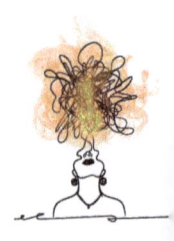

TODAY

The potential of a new day
It peaks through the curtains as I lay
Awake and burdened by yesterday
My regrets and fears on continuous replay

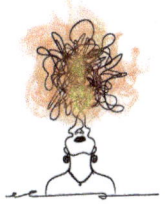

SPIRALLING INTO OBLIVION

I find myself spiralling out of control today
On a collision course towards my sanity
I let myself unwind last night
Let myself divest my carefully constructed self-control
I gave into hedonism, the moment
Dancing amongst the safety and company of good friends
And now I find myself in a fragile state of being
My recall of events patchy at best

I lost control, I took myself too far over that line I set for safety
And now my demons have resurfaced to taunt me fervently
Anxiety over what I may have said or done
Fear that I put myself at risk again
I try to piece together conversations had
They blur around the edges and fold in on themselves away from my sight

The more I try to seek them out
The more they disappear into the fog of my brain
My stomach lurches every which way
It knots itself within itself
Wringing out every last drop of rational thought with each minute that passes

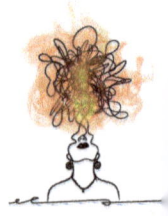

My twisted memory
My warped mind
My inner saboteur
My upside down logic

All rational thought leaves my being
And I continue to spiral
It's never ending
This need to punish myself
For having a little fun and letting go for just a little while

I try to centre myself again
Waiting for the processing to reach its natural end
Wishing I had some sort of filter
Hoping that next time I can enjoy myself without the fear of spiralling into oblivion
I sink to the floor exhausted at this fight with myself
Just one battle in the overall war
As I fight for myself against myself once more

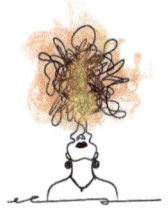

UNTITLED

Resolute between my truths
My half truths
That is where you will find me

Nestled between my white lies
My worst lies
That is where you will despise me

Intertwined in my memories
My daydreams
That is where you will think of me

Uncertain in my present
My future
That is where you will see me

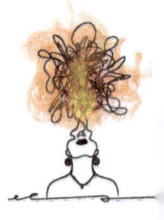

ACCEPTANCE

I am an eternal people pleaser
Determined to stay within your good graces
And when I find that I have lost your favour
I compromise myself to regain that spot
Each time I lose a little of myself
To become the person that I believe you want to see and know
I fight my moral compass
Just to gain your acceptance of me
For no matter how brief
And I resent myself for needing it so much

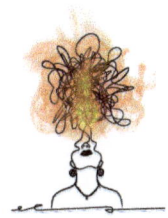

FROM THE SEDUCED TO THE SEDUCER

I lost myself in your smile
As the lights faded into memory
Diving into your eyes
I tried to find your ocean floor
Starstruck by your beauty
And seduced by those mellow tones
I found myself
And you held me tight in your gaze
Feelings of calm
Between those delirious words
I had found myself a safe haven
You had found a distraction
Both knowing it wouldn't last
An unusually comforting thought
Consequences unknown, forgotten
Unwanted, not said
I can't say that
You will ever think of me again
But the memory burns stronger
And hope knows what lust feels

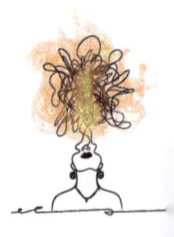

GHOSTED BY YOU

I thought that smile was just for me
I guess I was wrong, now I see
I feel a fool, I've been waiting for you
You've been radio silent, me without a clue
A knife in my back, pushed in deep
Shame and worry, been losing me sleep
I've done what I can, only this left to do
Block your number, redact it too
Lock this door and melt the key
In the fire of my flames, as I set myself free

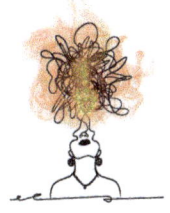

LAST DANCE

I count one, the music does start
A fluttering sound of my beating heart
I count two, he pulls me near
My blood pulsates, I smell his fear
I count three, before we glide and sway
I wait for the cue, till then we stay
I count four, we move to the beat
Our bodies lock, we're feeling the heat

I count five, finishing each step
Our eyes meet, intense contact is kept
I count six, rhythmic movements speak words
The music echoes all that is heard
I count seven, he shows me the way
The language of love has a lot to say
I count eight, as the tempo slows
The face is taut, the heart still glows
I count nine, he loosens his grip
We move into position, my body he dips
I count ten, the music has stopped
We end the dance, my hand is dropped

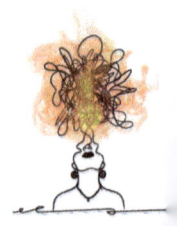

REFLECTIONS, REGRETS, REPOSE

I see what we have become
Comfortable, habitual, a ritual of domesticity
I yearn for those halcyon days
Full of passion, vernal longings, a dance of getting to know and love you

I feel us plateau and drift
Our accustomed roles providing assuaging complacency
I remember the vows we made to each other
Resolute and uncompromisingly we promised each other the world, our futures, unreservedly

I learn to steel myself against your barbs
But your litany of my shortcomings pierces my resolve
I ache to feel cherished by you again
The realisation that this can never be cuts deep

I remain trapped in abiding duty
And we continue to plateau and drift
Plateau and drift
Plateau and drift

A glimpse of what we had falls into obscurity
I lay myself at your mercy
Knowing the end is inevitable
But I quietly and stubbornly refuse to relinquish hope

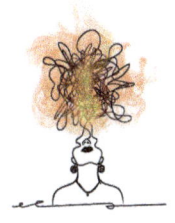

LEFT ON A READ RECEIPT

I keep staring at the last message I sent you
Waiting to see those three dots flashing
Or see you typing in our chat
But it has been 21 days
21 days since you last acknowledged me
The last exchange foretold nothing of what was to transpire
That we would end up here
With my messages hanging on a read receipt

I thought we knew each other well enough
To speak up when something was wrong
To talk through our issues together
But alas, I've become a victim of your absence
And I seem to be the only one
Well I can only assume that

As of 10 days ago you blocked me on social media
But not before I saw you hanging out with someone new
A face I didn't recognise, a name never mentioned previously
Her arm gripping you tightly
Her smile possessive
You looking into her eyes the way you used to with mine

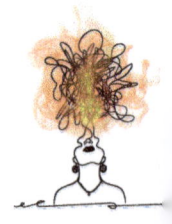

But of course the explanation could be perfectly innocent, right?
I shouldn't jump to conclusions
Well, I did that already didn't I!
From days 2 to 4
I ran through all possible reasons that you couldn't or wouldn't reply

From days 5 to 19
I listed all the possible things I did wrong
From days 19 to now
I have wallowed in regret
Because on days 6, 9, 12, 13 and 14…and 17

I messaged you again just to see if you would read them
And you did, you read every single one I sent
I might leave it one more day just in case…

…I think, as I scroll through photos of us, together, happy, smiling, enjoying each other

After all it's been 6 glorious months of getting to know everything about each other…

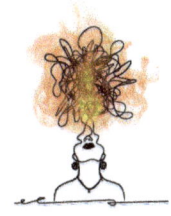

SUBMISSION

I stand here naked in contemplation
    My skin itches and burns
        Your eyes sear every inch of me
            I feel the scrutiny of your gaze
                I hear the judgement in your voice
                    I taste your dominance on my tongue
                        As you mark me for your own
                            I sense my punishment will be exacting
                                And I submit willingly, *but with regret*

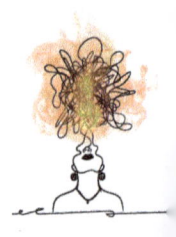

NOT MY OWN SELF

I begin to write but realise the handwriting isn't mine
I don't remember saying those words
And the Dictaphone is on pause
This scripted part a vague memory of something seen on tv
All my feelings fed in
Like an old computer game played to death
With game over I realise
It was all you
The tv remote fixed in your hand

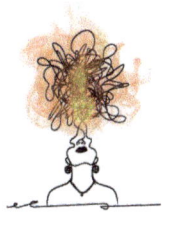

A CHANCE MEETING

Once more I found myself in his eyes
A flicker of feeling
A smile of remembrance
Lust shot through my naked veins
My body aches for his touch
A meeting of bodies
A glimmer of passion
Exhilaration encircled my sensory core
He wanted me to relive the past
A moment of hesitation
A jolt to my brain
My mind gracefully declined

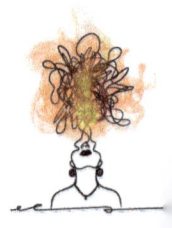

MANSPLAINING

I struggle for space as you make no room
You label me fragile, but you shouldn't assume
Once I carve out a niche I can call my own
You take it from me, as you claim your throne
When I voice an opinion, you shut me down
You scared I that want to take your crown
Now when I start to speak, I find you muted my mic
You further rig the game, so I lose each fight
As I rattle the cage that you've put me in
You take from me what I fought to win
But I refuse to play your vicious game
I'll win back myself and I'll bear no shame

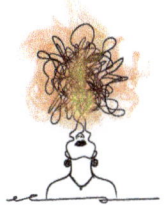

BLUES BAR RENDITION

She sings a tale of woe to an empty, smoky bar
No one cares for her sorrow, trouble, strife or terrible pain
But still she sings till silence is bought by her tired chords
The violinist snaps his bow in protest and sympathy
The piano takes it to the bridge to fill the silence, join the cause
The waitress pours another drink waiting for the closing bell
Still her pain is strummed and beaten out with force
All comes down to the final verse as the last bar seals her fate
She pauses to take a breath before the final protest of innocence
However, the trumpet takes the lead and silence is screeched at last

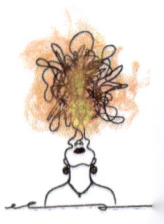

PRESENT

We are forced to recognise our current affinity
Neither of us wants to acknowledge its present state
Living in the memories of what we used to have
Planning for salvation
We discuss what will be
Compromising our spousal objectives
Hoping that we will restore our happenstance
We quietly acquiesce
That the present will heal us
But only if we face it together with fortitude

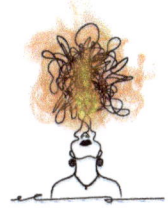

DEAR...

Dear Mother, you couldn't listen
When I tried to tell you, something was wrong
I was screaming in silence like a noise in a void
Space was bending you the other way
And the spotlight missed my cue

Dear teachers, you were all so kind
You kept me from drowning
You gave me sanctuary in those years
And I am forever grateful

Dear therapist, I lied, I wasn't strong
To talk for an hour became my sanctuary
But it never mattered, I was still trapped
And I couldn't find my way out of the darkness

Dear friend, I took it out on you
I'm sorry, please tell me what to do
You couldn't understand but tried
And you were always by my side

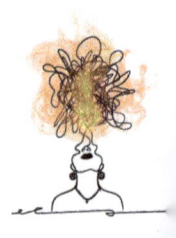

Dear me, forget the past, its done and gone
You love the life you have now
To be truthful it was always meant to be this way
It helped shape the woman I am today

To whom it may concern…
Don't take me at face value, get to know the real me
It might surprise us both what you will find
Beneath the perfect, where the words flow from my mind

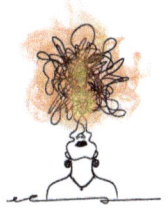

RELATIONSHIP GOALS

We skirt around the big issues
And obsess over the quick wins
We never set out our boundaries
Or learnt how to converse when it mattered
We interact between the things unsaid
Focusing on the trivia easier to speak
We circle back on old ground inevitably
And draw battle lines we will not cross
We hand each other platitudes vehemently
Waiting to see which ones stick tightly
We swop indignant glances, eyes full of disdain
One of us needs to draw a line
We need to break this perpetual game

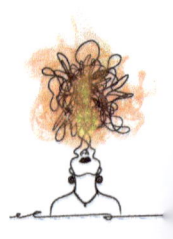

GOODBYE TO A LOYAL FRIEND

Go now dear friend
Its time
Go with your head held high
A stout heart and gentle touch
Its time now
Leave us all behind
Don't look back
Don't worry
Its time
Go now dear friend
We will meet on the other side

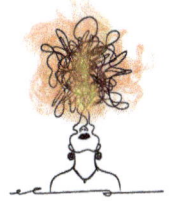

STALEMATE

I gave you my words
Admittedly a little late in the day
I tried to explain why they were ordered that way
I think you have read them
I can tell by your eyes
The way that they cannot quite meet mine for long
I can tell by your words
The way they skirt round the topic
But never quite reach it directly
You ask me about the periphery of it all
Clearly wanting me to know that you are interested
But we cannot seem to bridge the divide that sits between us
We talk in circles about the mundane
A safety blanket for both of us
I guess this is another in a long line of stalemates
The way that we have always communicated
Always missing the point unless in anger
For I am not going to ask
And I leave it up to you to tell

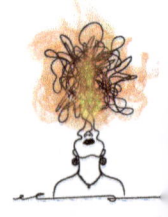

THE WAY WE CONVERSE WITH EACH OTHER

I stand under the spray
Punch drunk by our recent encounter
Your words landing square on my jaw
I cannot recall how it started
But I can still feel how it finished
My emotions black and blue
All I asked for was a little respect
Some consideration of how your decisions affect me
But you are so used to getting things your way
As I learnt to compromise to keep the peace
This has become my go to move
The middle ground has now become the battle ground
Where I fight to fix my boundaries
Where you dictate the terms of my surrender
Throwing my words back at me to protect your own insecurities
I have learnt your strategies
I plan my next move
I dig in, refusing to give up ground
It isn't pretty, but it's a start
I promise myself that I shall no longer be the martyr
I tend my wounds, the water cleansing everything
Whilst I consider my position carefully
And I prepare myself for the negotiations to come

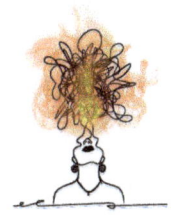

HIDING FROM THE DARKNESS OF YOU

I thought I had found the perfect hiding place
An alcove at the back of the room
Screened by something pink and gaudy
Consumed by fear and the need to protect myself
A record player in my head on repeat with some kitsch band I thought might sing away my woes
But you found me
I trapped with no way out
A deer in headlights
My throat tightened
My words stuck inside
I steeled myself
An attempt to make myself a difficult target
But still you came
I didn't think you'd ever be this way
I thought I knew you better
And as you tried to take what wasn't yours
As you tried to claim something of me that I would never freely give you

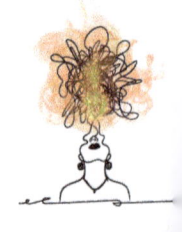

I found my voice
Just as your touched me
I screamed
Loudly
GET YOUR HANDS OFF ME!
You weren't expecting that
I tried not to sob
You backed off as you heard footsteps coming towards us
And all at once you were gone
But I couldn't sigh in relief
Tears streaking down my face
I hugged myself tight
Wondering if I would ever be safe from you again

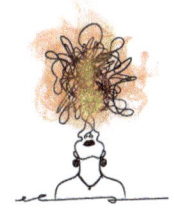

PROVOCATION

We lasted 4 days, 18 hours, 30 minutes and 24 seconds in our blissful little world
That was until you baited me once again
Drove those needle-sharp words into my gut
Doubling me over in shock and pain
Twisting me over until I gasped for breath
You knew I wouldn't be able to hold back
That if forced into a corner, I'd defend myself, my words at the ready
You pushed all the right buttons
Let me fire off those syllables
Direct hits to your head
And then you make a show of being wounded as you got what you wanted
An excuse to paint me in gothic horror
To give you carte blanche
As you think on how you will use this
I realise I have been sucker punched again
I gave you what you wanted
I compromised my composure
And now I will reap the consequences

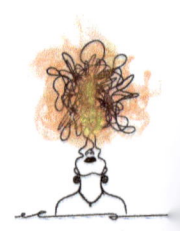

WAR PAINT

I look into the bathroom mirror
Mapping out how I will mark my defences
I must look fierce tonight
My visage must hide my suffering
Nobody can see the cracks that traverse my countenance
I set out my palette
I line up my brushes
I close my eyes and muster my courage
I will my hand to steady
Inhaling, I see the effect I wish to achieve
And I start to paint myself
All the time I paint, I whisper
They don't deserve to know the real you
Give them of yourself only what you trust them to keep safe
Keep all the rest of you for those who love you for who you really are
Remember that you are beautiful, inside and out
Your smile will light up the room
As I put the final coat of lipstick on
I take in my war paint, as flawless as I can hope for
I see a warrior queen before me
I feel strong
I feel battle ready
Smiling, I turn off the light
Put on my heels
And head to the front door

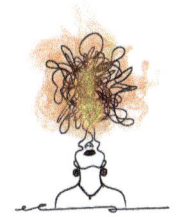

KEEPING MYSELF SAFE FROM THE DARKNESS OF YOU

I could never have guessed how things would turn out between us
From the comfortable intimacy of friendship
To the fear and anxiety of each phone call and text message
Which would manifest as soon as the screen displayed your name
I still cannot decipher whether you realised what you were doing
With the intimidation and fear you caused
Or whether you thought I was playing coy
Encouraging you to become bolder in your attempts
I tried to reason with you, set you straight
And when that proved fruitless
I tried to ignore you
Hoped that I could ghost you away
But nothing worked

It wasn't until you
Tried to possess me
Tried to undress me
I knew that you weren't oblivious to the distress of me

That I realised my only protection would be distance
That I had to cut those ties

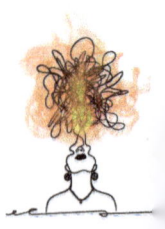

But you wouldn't accept that
And the last time we coexisted in the same space
You made a public apology for your "behaviour"
Tried to reconcile all you had done, publicly
Where you knew I couldn't
I wouldn't cause a scene
So, when you embraced me to seal the apology
Your grip like a vice

Still trying to possess me
Clearly still wanting to undress me
Knowing that this would distress me

I froze, stiffened awkwardly
All I wanted to do was claw at you to release me
Scream at you to leave me alone
I tried not to shake
Or sob, or show any weakness
I went along with your game
Put up my façade
And once I could get away, I ran
Trying to put as much distance between us as I could
Knowing that this would be the only way
That I could keep myself safe from the darkness of you

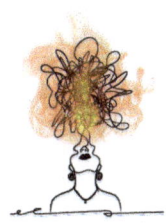

HOW FAR I FELL INTO DARKNESS

I didn't realise how far I had
                    fallen
                        into
                            the
                                darkness
At least not until I bumped my head as I was coaxed from under my desk
Worried eyes giving me the once over
Checking for obvious signs of injury
Not that they would find any as it was all internal
All deep-seated self-loathing and shame and fear
The smell of it all burning in my nostrils
I couldn't look anyone in the eye
That's when I knew I hit
                    rock
                        bottom
All I wanted to do was curl into a ball
Or retreat to the darkest corner I could find
Anything to stop the eyes on me
            Even though they were filled with kindness and worry
                            They burned my soul
                Made me realise how unpretty I had become
            Then at once I was stating my case to the Doctor
                        Not quite meeting her gaze
                    Unable to form coherent sentences

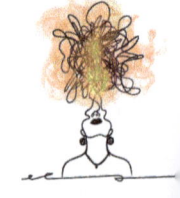

Pointing to the lowest scores on the paper
A test to assess my current state of mind
Then I realised I was still
                    falling
                          to
                              rock
                                  bottom
That I was questioning my will to survive
To stay alive and kicking
All I wanted was for it all to stop
To exist in the void between the living and the dead
That quiet place where I wouldn't feel a thing
                              Now I had hit rock bottom
                              I admitted my shameful thoughts
                      Not quite being able to articulate the cause
                          Wanting to keep some secrets back
That's when the pills were pushed into my hands
The ones to regulate my emotions
These would bring the everlasting nausea
The ones to help me sleep
These would leave a metallic taste
                Now I would learn to crawl along rock bottom
                              Caught in a fugue state
             Hungry as hell but unable to stomach a morsel
This is when I realised rock bottom was such a long way down in
                                      the darkness
So, I started to cling to the sides of the abyss
And slowly drag myself up one day at a time

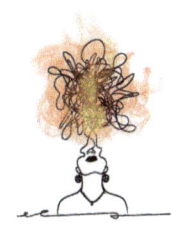

NO SUITOR WAS RIGHT FOR ME

I tried so hard to conform
To be what was expected of me
To be the perfect, pretty young thing
Husband hunting to fulfil society's expectations of me
I tried so hard to find the perfect suitor
But always chose the wrong ones
The power hungry types
The break your heart types
The won't respect you types

Although some were right for other reasons as they were
The commitment phobe types
The good time types
The long distance til it fizzles types
I learnt all about
Cruel love
Physical love
Requited love
Longing
Desire
Shame and power and control
Breaking hearts and unfulfillment

But I never found true love
I never found the comfort of intimacy
Only the comfort of being left or running away

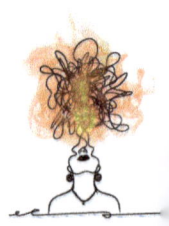

For me, it was always rehearsed
Always a performance
Sometimes I even convinced myself it was real
I was always settling
Thinking that this was all I was worth
Trying to find the best of worst I could have

Hoping that the sick feeling in my stomach wouldn't give me away
Wishing I could be the real me
Wanting to understand why I couldn't just be normal

But for all the bad times there were the good ones, happy times
And whilst I knew that no fairytale would come true for me
Each suitor taught me that I'd only be happy once I was free to be me
So, I thank them all for that

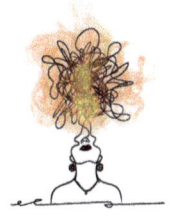

CRASH AND BURN

Today I want to tear my skin from my flesh and bones
I claw at myself again and again trying to find purchase
Waiting to find a spot to sink my fingernails into
Everything burns white hot, acrid and smoking

Nobody warned me that it would be like this
That both my actions and inactions could cause so much pain, so everlasting
As I obsess about what I should have done
What I could have done
All those options crowding my mind
It's all swirling and adding fuel to the fire of my regrets
My anxiety and self-loathing rallying to the cause
They conspire against me, torture my mind
Keep me in a heightened state of disquietude
Haunting my waking dreams, my every thoughts
Until it is just me

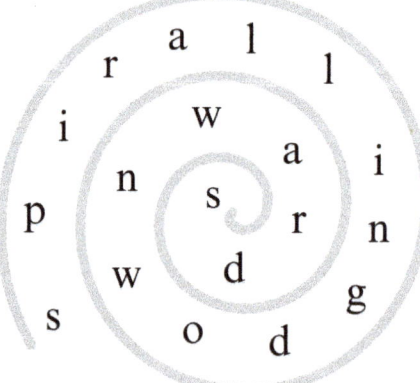

spiralling inwards towards sadness

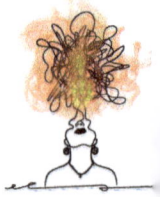

Like a runaway train on a collision course
I can see it coming clear as day
But I have run out of escape routes
I am forced to watch it all in slow motion
The exact point at which I implode
As my mind cannot take anymore
To protect itself and me, it shuts down
Throwing me into that apathetic state again
I become listless, torpid and inert

Fighting myself to function with a smile or even any care at all
I paint on my fake smile, and find my fake happy voice
Hoping that this latest episode won't last too long
That I can find myself again and carry on

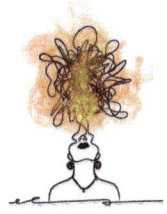

WHERE I HIDE MY TEARS

I try not to let it destroy me
The pain of failing to get your approval

So I hide it
In the smiles I flash everybody's way
In the love and support I give to the others I care for
In the words of wisdom, I impart when asked
I hide my tears more often than I would like
In the car before I reach each destination
In the freshness of the morning, as I walk the waggy tails
In the nib of my pen as I write these words

And I dwell upon this too much
In my morning shower, my head beneath the spray
In between the voice of the cuckoo at each hour of the day
In the silent moments before I sleep and as I wake

So, I tell myself each day that

I only need my own approval to be happy
I only need to be proud of me to validate all that I achieve
I only want my cheerleaders to stand next to me

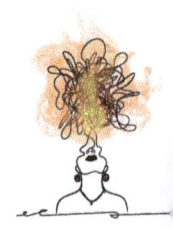

THE EVERLASTING TORMENT OF YOUR WORDS

I do not feel the bravery that people confer on me
As I write the words of my history, my present, my pain

My eyes only see the shame of what I cannot achieve
My ears only hear the rejections ringing loud
My heart only feels each time I wasn't enough

I try to steer towards the positivity of others
Let them be my North Star

But the wounds were cut deep, a thousand times over
And I cannot stop myself from going back for more
Like a moth to the flame
Like the need for water in the desert

I am still bound in your chains
Even though I broke through them years ago

It's the ghost of hope that always pulls me back in
And the desire for survival that brings me back to life again

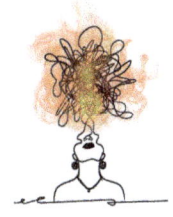

WHEN THE WATER OVERWHELMED

In the last ten plus days I have picked up my pen several times
It has hovered over the page waiting for my emotions to stream
But nothing coherent came
Instead I was a pressure cooker of emotions which boiled just under the surface of my entire being

I needed to keep them in check
Rein them in to focus on my role
To be what was needed
To do what was expected and necessary

At times I lost that tight control
The weight of all those emotions seeping through that veil between emotional control and chaos

My frustrations fuelling my anger
My heartbreak fuelling my grief

At times it felt like the dam had burst so I would not be able to function

My exhaustion doubling my emotional intensity
My insomnia doubling my need to do more than I could

But what I forgot was that I cannot boil the sea
I cannot decant the water with only any egg cup
I can only do my best

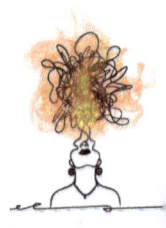

I know that I did my best during these days
I know that I put everything else before myself to do what needed to be done

However, it would never have been enough
I hope that one day that this gets through to me

Until then I try not to layer the pressure of responsibility and heartbreak upon myself

Stitched together by my emotions which weigh heavy on my weary shoulders

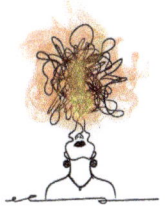

STUCK

The rut is deep and I am at the bottom
Trying to work out how to free myself
This mind prison, with walls closing in
The claustrophobia threatening with every inhale of breath

I find myself stuck
Circling the void I find myself in
Stuck at the edge of the darkness
Screaming without sound

My head pounding
My eyes squeezed shut
Wishing that I could be anywhere but here

As the darkness threatens
I slowly take another pass of the void
Hoping to find a way to break free

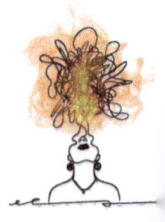

I KNEW THAT THE DARKNESS WAS BACK

I knew as the sick feeling in my stomach grew
I knew as my nightmares got worse and more frequent
I knew when I lost interest in my favourite things
I knew when I avoided eye contact with everyone else
I knew when the manic episodes increased
I knew that the darkness was back
I knew that as the monochrome took over
I knew as the ringing in my ears increased
I knew as it became difficult to break the inertia in me
I knew that I needed help
I knew that if I didn't get help, I would slowly disappear

So I admitted that I wasn't ok
To myself
To those closest to me
I dialled the number
Afraid of what I would have to say
But relieved that I had done this today

Now starts the climb from rock bottom once more

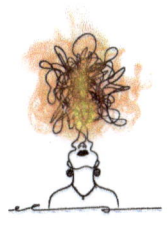

CHEMICAL SUBMISSION

If you lean closer towards me and look into my eyes
You will find unshed tears, frozen in time
Caught at the moment they were about to fall down

As my emotions began to creep over the precipice and into the everlasting darkness
They were cast into stone by the chemistry of balance
Smoothing the extremes I feel
Wrangling the outliers until they were reined into the centre point
Equilibrium on prescription

I don't feel in control of my feelings
But they behave for now as they are muted
Quietened, chemically altered into submission

I am emotionally discombobulated, feeling all yet nothing
A temporary measure it is hoped

So I can regain control of my mind once more

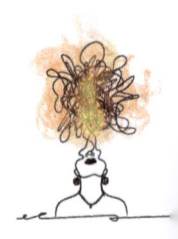

UP AND DOWN, AGAIN AND AGAIN

Wings clipped for my protection
My senses dulled
I, full of emotions
My body wracked with unwanted movements
I experience it all in slow motion
Just when I think I'm beginning to feel more settled
The tempo flips
I find myself fully awake
Aware of every little sound
Every sensation heightened
I flinch react as I'm breathing
Eyes rapidly searching for the threat
Mind entering into overdrive
Heart rate competing with itself
Just when I think my body cannot take the pace
That my mind will implode as it calculates all the variables
The tempo flips again
Each hour is like this
As I wait for the medicine to kick in
I wait for even tones
I wait for the chemical equilibrium
I wait for peace of mind
Until then I strap myself in for the unwanted theme park ride
Hoping that it finishes soon

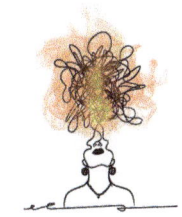

BREAKING FREE OF THE DARKNESS ONCE MORE

I sit here trying to reverse my spiral
The weight of responsibility hanging heavy
My emotions black and blue despite time and distance
Nightmares have plagued my sleep for the last week
Each one more intense than the last
They have me trapped in a feedback loop
My days feel like I am wading through quicksand
Slowly being sucked deeper into my spiral with each step
My skin raw, begging for me to rip the flesh with my nails or something sharper
Anything to cut out the pain and misery
The little voice reappears in the back of my head taunting me with whispers
"Failure"
"Useless"
"Why didn't you do better"
Then comes the worst whispers of all
"They would do better without you"
I take to my bed, curling in a ball
Hoping sleep will help
Wondering how I had let those words back in
When I thought I had vanquished that little voice
This is when I realise how low I have become
Caught on the verge of catatonia, as I close in on myself
My anxiety heightened

Restless but every reaction is slowed to an almost stop
Autopilot kicks in
Trapped in negativity, I fight to regain control
And fight I must because this is not where I want to be
I have worked too hard to let myself disappear
I have clawed myself out of the abyss so many times before
I won't let this take me down in the darkness
I just need something to break the feedback loop
A kickstart to remind me of how far I have come

I feel you come towards me unsure of how I will react
As you ask to kiss me, I feel myself pull back, considering myself unworthy
But as your lips touch mine I feel your love
It's as if I am sleeping beauty
Who has been given true love's kiss
My eyes are suddenly wide open
My lungs are full of air which I slowly release
A warmth spreads throughout my limbs

I smile slowly knowing that the spiralling has ceased
That I am coming round from my stupor
And I have broken free of the darkness once more

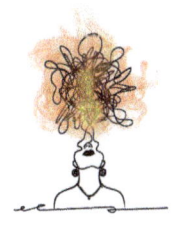

THE DARKNESS HAUNTS ME STILL

It once took me 274 days
To climb from the bottom of the abyss
A medicated sticky plaster
Patching me up as best it could
Whilst I screamed silently in my head
Punch drunk on chemicals
Which left me emotionless
Famished
Sick to my stomach
Heavy limbed
Needing to wear a mask of perfect, which I struggled to keep up
As I got halfway through those days of climbing
A new challenge befell me
The time to wean me off that plaster
It wasn't an ideal plan
For I couldn't rip it off
I had to slowly peel it bit by bit
I had to strip back myself to the bone
Each week would allow me to feel a little more
And with that came the pain and the panic
The dual antagonists I battled
The fear of falling again renewed
As my awareness improved

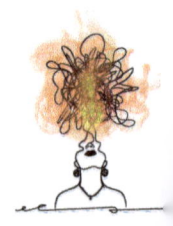

The Breaking of Me | Lisa Scovell-Strickland

The shame seeped its way back in
All those other emotions flooded back
Fuelled by my anxiety that I couldn't cope
That the darkness would shroud me once more
And this time it would grip harder than before
But to my surprise I didn't fall
At times I sunk to my knees
But I got back up
It wasn't pretty, I like a new born
I fumbled, staggered
Like drunk dancing when you think you know the moves
But I kept going
Getting stronger everyday
Now as I look back to then, I see
I see that the darkness was still there
Lingering in me, clinging to my soul
Waiting for me to weaken
Haunting me day and night
Now I know that it still attacks
Still tries to drag me back down to rock bottom
However, I won't let it take me
For I see it coming
I arm myself well
And I banish it back to black

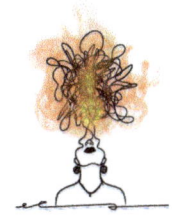

THE BITTER TASTE OF SLEEP

I find myself awake again
Unable to calm my mind
Thoughts raging, my body restless
Obsessing about things in the past
Worrying about things yet to come
I try counting sheep
I try counting backwards
I try everything I can think of
Nothing brings the rest I desperately need

Reluctantly I reach for a chemical cure
The prescription freshly filled
I choke the required dose down with resignation and water
Knowing it won't be long now till I drift into slumber
Dreading the after effects that await me in the morning
That metallic taste that lingers all day
The head fog that makes me feel numb
The heaviness of my limbs
The feeling of defeat because I needed to medicate again

But in this moment I only focus on relief
My eyes grow tired
My body finally still
My mind quietening
As I finally fall into a dreamless slumber

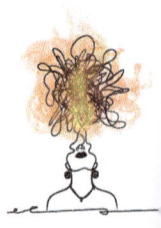

HAPPENSTANCE NO MORE

I cleaved myself open to oust the pain we left each other
Thinking this would be enough to bridge the divide
Hoping it would heal the wound, dampen my guilt
But all it has done is put us at polar opposites
Needing a satellite to communicate
Requiring the right orbit to activate the connection
I thought I had paid my penance
Washed away my sins of before
Brokered a peace to last us to the end of our days
However, all I have done is subvert the happenstance we had
Laid bare truths that couldn't stay hidden
If you have taken my truths personally
I don't blame you, I just want to know why
Is it because I walk my own path now?
Or is it because you are no longer the brightest stars in my night sky?

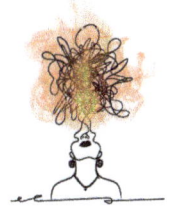

THE GHOST IN THE HALLWAY MIRROR

I stand in the hallway peering into the looking glass
A sobering view returns to me
I want to feel alive again
To feel the surge of life course through my veins
But I am weak and numb
Caught in a torpid state
I long for a loving touch to ignite my soul
Hoping that it will be yours
Wishing that you can see the need in me
Wanting you to set me free
Could you do that for me?
Will you resurrect me?
Can you save me from my despair?
And as my eyes flick from the hallway mirror and back again
The ghost of me looks back weakly smiling
Whispering to me
I am trying to be everything that you need
I am fighting for you every day
Slowly I raise my hand to my cheek
Brushing away the tears as they fall
Cupping my cheek, I whisper back
I am learning to love you
Be patient I am fighting for you too
Every day, hour, minute and second
For as long as it takes
No matter what

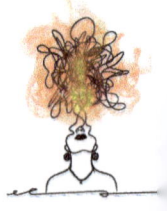

THE WORDS IN MY HEAD

Sometimes my words escape me
I find it difficult to catch them
As they run out of my mind
Before I can put them on the page
But it is the words buried deep inside me
The ones that refuse to be coaxed out
These are the ones that scare me
For once they surface
Once they let themselves be known
I know that I will have to deal with them
I won't be able to ignore them for long
As they tell my darkest truths
My inner fears, my deepest desires
They let themselves be known
The loudest whisper in my thoughts
Like a record on repeat
They sound the tolling of the bell
Waiting to be recognised and recorded
As I scribble them frantically
I see that these will be my best words
But that they strip me naked
My truths inked into my skin
In works of art
Waiting to be read, desperate to be seen
Certain to ruin me, Break me, destroy me
Setting fire to the old me
And allowing me to be reborn again

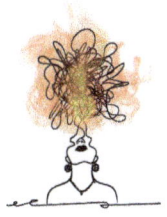

AFTER THE WORLD REOPENED

When the darkness struck again I barely noticed
I was too invested in the support of others
My time divided between supporting the living and caring for the dead
This left little space for me to take care of myself
I tried to but took the wrong approach
I bottled those feelings up
Letting my anxiety lead
It served me well in keeping on top of it all
But all at once I noticed that I had fallen
Not quite to rock bottom but a fair way down
What I noticed most was my anger
Burning bright and hair triggered
I had to swallow it as it often rose high in my throat
My tongue becoming forked and negative
Hurtful thoughts ready to be voiced upon command
Sometimes they just slipped out
And as the world reopened for business
I noticed too, the fear of the front door
Leaving the house to face the outside world
A suffocating feeling in my chest whenever I had to use it for anything other than exercise

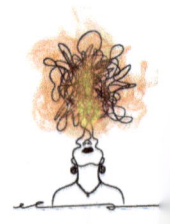

And I noticed the pain of seeing so much suffering and being unable to fix it
Bewildering that I couldn't even fix myself with my usual tools
The garden had become my sanctuary
The dog walks had become my release

But I had to force myself to do so much more

To reconnect without a screen

To convene without focusing on the fear

To be comfortable in the company of others

Each day had its challenges
As I struggled to reintegrate
All the time wondering if I would ever be myself again

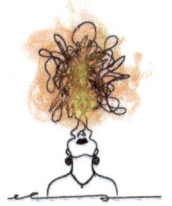

THE BATHROOM MIRROR CRACKED

All used up and incomplete
I can't stand to look myself in my eyes
I don't recognise my face
A tableau of lies and deceit reenact my latest attempts to fit into this world
The fake happy soul I can be no more

My inner monologue is bursting to get free of my skin
Waiting for the cracks to form
To get the chance to expose the real me
Although I'm not sure what is real anymore
Where I begin or where the scripted me ends

I cannot take another day of self denial
It's killing me slowly
My soul being strangled with each breath I take
As I deny myself once more
Deny the core of me
Deny the best of me
Shroud myself in shame and dress up myself in the essence of something I think they want to see

But this only allows the atrophy to set in
As I let myself go, wither away
My brightness dimming
My colour fading to monochrome
Sucking the joy from my smile

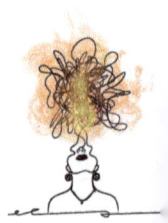

All I can do now is take that lipstick and paint my lips Ruby red
Hope that they don't notice the cracks

But I don't want to live like this, I hear myself say
A voice long since buried with a fury I thought I had lost
I want to fight for myself
The real me
The secret me
The best of me
I don't want to hide like this anymore

Looking at the mirror again
I see a crack appear
Hairline from left to right above my left eye
It travels towards my nose and down across my mouth
As it hits my neck I see a glimmer of light trying to push its way out
All bright and beautiful

There it is, that's the real me
The golden and the warmth that needs to be set free
As my smile widens, my fingers touch my cheek
I whisper thank f**k for that
Bathed in the light of me for the first time
As I realise that the bathroom mirror cracked, not me

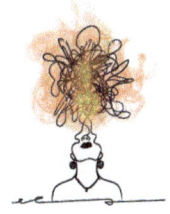

EXHAUSTION

I have never known weariness like this
Every muscle and bone harbouring that heavy feeling
From the tips of my toes to the follicles of my hair
Nothing escapes the heaviness, the pain of overuse
But I have not run a marathon, well not physically

This uncomfortable state results from decompression
The act of me letting everything I have been holding onto go
For every breakthrough has a cost
Each time I overcome a fear
Rewrite the narrative to positive
Take a brave step forward
Fight that anxiety
It leaves me breathless and fatigued

The journey from survival to sanctuary has been a long one
It hasn't been linear
I have backtracked
U-turned
Fallen and picked myself back up
And each one of these had added to my fatigue
At times I have turned numb
Mistaking my progress for flight from an unknown threat
Sometimes I froze unable to celebrate the success of getting this far

For no one tells you this part
That for every demon you vanquish
With every endorphin it releases to fill you with pride at your achievement it also exhausts you

As each layer of survival sheds slowly
Sometimes it is fleeting
Sometimes it lasts for days
As you struggle to maintain positivity
When it hurts to put one foot in front of another

But I don't resent this
I savour this exhaustion
Relish the heaviness of my limbs
For my progress is my salvation
An acknowledgment of all I have overcome
A testament to my refusal to give up
And when the exhaustion passes
I can say I survived
I conquered
I am alive
Ready to start on my own terms
In the direction that I want to go
With my future uncharted in front of me
Waiting to be discovered

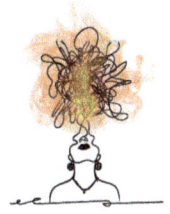

IN BETWEEN

I find myself between two worlds
A foot on either side of the divide
Feeling the pull of each gravity weighing heavy on my mind and body

The world to my left is my old life
A place where the girl I used to be resides
A world of missed opportunities

The shackles of all my pain waiting to ensnare me once more
I see now the reruns of my traumas being watched on the tv set
The lounge in which it is situated plays a merry tune to entice me to watch it back

A cold and foggy gloom envelopes this world like a horror movie I once owned on videocassette
The audio doesn't quite sync with the picture
And I realise that I no longer wear that skin, the shedding of it still feels new

The world to my right is the new life I have chosen for myself
The glorious technicolour striking a bold pose about the place
Everything looks and feels brand new

But as I look closer I realise it is all as it used to be
Now I see it all through fresh eyes

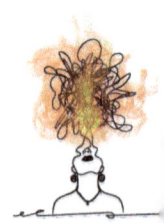

The itching of new skin distracts me from this notion

I feel a little uncomfortable in my new skin

I feel overwhelmed but in a good way

I am exhausted from the fight of having transformed myself anew

But as I look up to the dawn sky
My wings still aflame
I turn to the left to see the trail of ashes to the old world

Then I step to the right
Two feet firmly planted exactly where I want them to be
Watching the last vestiges of the world I came from
As it disappears from my view

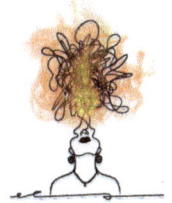

www.ingramcontent.com/pod-product-compliance
Lightning Source LLC
Chambersburg PA
CBHW061751070526
44585CB00025B/2861